I0489165

ANAL SEX :
THE SEXUAL ABUSE OF A NON SEXUAL ORGAN
with huge health risks INCLUDING STERILITY.

SEX IS FOR PROCREATION AND IT WAS NEVER INTENDED FOR RECREATION.

IF EVERYONE PRACTICES ANAL SEX FOR PLEASURE, HUMANS WILL HAVE ANOTHER SODOM AND GOMORRAH FATE AND THE END OF THE HUMAN RACE!

BY : S. ELLISS

Disclaimer:
 I write this book to emphasize the potential huge
health risks when engaging in any sexual activity
and especially anal sex. This book is for
information only and is not intended to offend any
one that has a different view, or preferences on
this controversial subject. Whatever consenting
adults are doing in the privacy of their home is their
business and it is nobody's else business to

interfere on what is going on in their bedrooms. However we seldom hear what's going in the privacy of peoples bedrooms but we often hear the scandals and sexual abuse, anal and otherwise of youngsters by sexual predators and that's the big problem and concern for the human society. Whether consensual ,coerced, or forced anal sex , if there is bleeding, pain or other health symptoms it is advisable to seek medical attention as soon as possible. Anal sexual activity consensual or otherwise can cause serious health problems and it is advisable to see your doctor for proper diagnosis and treatment.
The author.

S. ELLISS

Table of content

9)WHAT IS THE NORMAL NATURAL FUNCTION OF THE ANUS?

10)The pros and cons of anal sex.

A)The pros of anal sex, if any.

B)The cons of anal sexual activity.

11)Comparing the Sexual habits of humans to other animals.

12)Another dangerous human sexual practice is the Oral sex?

13)THE PURPOSE OF THE SEXUAL ACTIVITY FOR ALL LIVING CREATURES.

14)POTENTIAL HEALTH RISKS TO BOTH PARTIES OF ANAL SEX

15)THE ROLE OF CHURCH AND ANAL

SEXUAL ACTIVITY   OVER THE
YEARS.
THE CHURCH CLERGY HAVE BEEN
PREYING ON THE YOUNG for many years.

16)THE PEDOPHILES ARE PREYING ON THE
YOUNG.

17)SEX EDUCATION 101

a)Sex education at home
b)Sex education in schools

18)The distinction   between
   love and sex

19)There are five camps in the anal
sex saga .

20)THE COURT DECISION THAT ABOLISHED
THE LAW PROTECTING THE YOUNGSTERS
from anal sex.

Introduction :

In this book the author expresses his views on

this controversial subject, based on the anatomy and physiology of the human body , the laws of nature and the potential huge health risks of any sexual activity including anal sexual activity. Lets not forget what comes out of the anal canal, the feces which is full of pathogenic viruses and bacteria. Every part of the body has a specific function to do and the anus function is to control and expel the waste byproducts of digestion. The anus is not part of the sexual organs and was never intended to be used for any sexual activity. The sex organs are for reproduction and not for recreation. The sexual organs job is to reproduce offspring for the continuation of its kind and nothing else. The humans for some reason want to sexualize everything, including the anus, the mouth , and other parts of the body that have nothing to do with the sexual organs.. In all the animal kingdom , only humans are obsessed with sex and created billions of dollars industries for profit at the expense of the human body. The rest of the animal kingdom instantly know exactly what is the role of the sexual organs, for procreation and never for recreation. The animals follow their natural instinct to procreate but the humans ignore their natural instinct for the sake of pleasure.

This book is for information only and not intended

to offend anybody's else opinion or preferences. Everyone is entitle to his or her opinion and preferences as long as they do not intrude and harm other peoples rights , personal safety and integrity. Whatever consenting adults do in the privacy of their home it is their business and nobody's else. We seldom hear what is going on in the homes of consenting adults, and it is none of our business to pry OF WHAT THEY DO OR THE OR WHAT THEY DO NOT DO. . But there are always news On the radio, newspapers, and television about sexual abuse, anal and otherwise, not about consenting adults , but about vulnerable innocent youngsters and adults both male and females and I think that's where the problem for society is. There was news on television that a pastor sexually abused more than 19 youngsters and his victims now grown up men are suing him and taking him to court for the years of abuse. I think it is about time all these victims to speak up and take legal action against their abusers. The sexual abuse , anal or otherwise of youngsters, is causing physical and psychological problems that scars them for life.

Years after their abuse, they still have physical and psychological problems and sometimes with catastrophic results. So , the practice of anal sex by consenting adults in the privacy of their homes is of no concern to society , but the sexual use and abuse of innocent non consenting persons it is of great concern to society.

The anus was never intended for any sexual activity , its main natural function is to control and expel the end waste product of digestion, called feces. Any sexual activity involving the anus has major health risks which we are going to explore later on.

WHAT IS ANAL SEX ANYWAY?

Anal sex is the penetration of the male or female anus by the male penis or any other object. Many people, whether they are heterosexual, gay, homosexuals or bisexual are willingly, coerced or forced to have anal sex. Anal sexual activity used to be practiced only by homosexual men, but in recent years , mainly due to misinformation in the sex education in schools , the anal sexual activity is spreading against the females as well, and that's very dangerous for women and society. Women were created by the all mighty god to produce babies and not to be used or abused as sex toys for pleasure.

Men used to prefer women with a tight vagina and when their vagina was stretched from overused or by giving birth to babies , some men were looking for another woman for a tight vagina and so on. Now a days they are looking for a tight anus even when a vagina is available. When that tight anus is not tight anymore they are looking for another tight anus to ruin no matter if it is a male or female anus. And that is a serious health problem, considering what comes out of the anus, the feces. The human feces is full of pathogenic germs which can cause serious infections. These infections can cause life threatening diseases and sterility to both men and women. If this trend continues, and everybody is practicing anal sex and people become sick and sterile you can understand that humans will eventually disappear from the face of the earth like the dinosaurs . The end of the human race will come because people they forgot that sex was for procreation and was never intended for recreation. The proponents for anal sex are talking about sexual pleasure, more sexual pleasure and nothing else. They even try to intimidate those that are concerned about such practice or are opposing their views.

People should consider the pros and cons before embarking in any adventurous and highly risky situation in which their lives and their health can be in serious danger. Anal sex can expose its participants to two principal dangers: a) infections due to the high number of infectious viruses and bacteria found in the human stool and b)of course the physical damage to the anus and rectum due to their fragility.

Repetitive penetrative anal sex may result in the anal sphincters to become weakened, which may cause rectal prolapsed, rectal perforation or affect the ability to hold in feces ,a condition known as fecal incontinence .

Potential Health risks such as sterility and infections for both men and women :

Rao kamini in his book " principles and practice of assisted reproductive technology" writes; "Unprotected anal sex is a risk factor for formation of antisperm antibodies (ASA) in the recipient. In some people, ASA may cause autoimmune infertility.[90] Antisperm antibodies impair fertilization, negatively affect the implantation process and impair growth and development of the embryo.[91][90] "

Kamini A. Rao

- Dr. Kamini A. Rao is a pioneer in the field of Assisted Reproduction in India. She has specialized in reproductive endocrinology and ovarian physiology.

kamini's findings are troublesome , because women and men can become sterile and unable to have babies , from practicing anal sex. That is a serious danger to humans' existence and can cause another Sodom and Gomorrah destruction by the all mighty nature.

Unprotected receptive anal sex (with an HIV positive partner) is the sex act most likely to result in HIV transmission. Other infections that can be transmitted by unprotected anal sex are human papillomavirus (HPV) ,which can increase the risk of anal cancer, typhoid fever, amoibiasis, Chlamydia, E. coli infections, gonorrhea, hepatitis A ,B and C, herpes simplex, salmonellas, shigella, syphilis and other infections.

Considering all the dangers and health risks to the participants of anal sex , one should wonder out loud , why anyone in his right mind would want to participate in such a highly risky sexual activity. Is the sexual pleasure worthy of loosing your health and getting sick and even your life? ?

Anyone in his or her right mind should think twice before embarking in such a risky sexual adventure. But then again humans are unpredictable with the choices they make, like the drug use and abuse, smoking, alcohol and other poor choices which harm the human body, but they still do it anyway .

HISTORY

THE SODOM AND GOMORRAH STORY.

The destruction of the cities Sodom and Gomorrah as a punishment for practicing anal sex by the all mighty god occurred long time ago somewhere in the middle east.

Many centuries ago there were these two cities in the middle east near the present state of Israel. The name of those cities were Sodom and Gomorrah and their inhabitants had the peculiar habit of practicing anal sex. They were obsessed with the anal sex and they wanted everyone to have anal sex. As the story goes, god was very angry about their unnatural choice and he sent two angels to investigate what was going on. The two angels dressed as ordinary men, went to the house of Abraham's nephew Lot who was the only one in those cities not practicing anal sex. Lot and his family lived in Sodom. Lot took the two angels to his home , fed them and arranged for their overnight stay. Then all the men of the city surrounded Lot's house and asked "Where are the two men who came to visit you tonight? Bring them out to us so that we can have anal sex with them." (Genesis 19:5, NIV). Lot offered them his two young virgin daughters to have sex with them instead, but they refused that offer, demanding to have anal sex with the two newcomer men. As the story goes, god was so furious with the abnormal behavior of the men of Sodom and Gomorrah, that he destroyed both Sodom and Gomorrah and spared only Lot , his wife and two daughters from the total destruction of those two sin cities. Lot's wife was curious about the destruction and when they were leaving the city , she looked back to see what was happening .God was angry with her and turned her into a pile of salt , so the story goes.

That's how the story ends with the destruction of those two sin cities, Gomorrah and Sodom, by the mighty god because of their unnatural ways of anal sex. And that's why anal sex is often referred to as SODOMY, from that long lost and destroyed city Sodom. To this day nobody knows where the exact location of those cities is because the destruction was so devastating and complete. Ever since that time, humans were so afraid that god might punish them if they engaged in any anal sexual activity that they made laws against (SODOMY) anal sex punishable by the local human laws. Those laws survived over the centuries until the recent years when some courts made local rulings abolishing the laws against anal sexual practice. We are going to examine some of those rulings to see what effects will have on people and the future of human society.

The story of Sodom and Gomorrah was the result of the reckless behavior of the inhabitants of those cities. whether the destruction was due to direct divine intervention or the direct result of diseases from the many pathogenic viruses and bacteria which are present in the feces, is not clear.

The people of that time did not know anything about viruses and bacteria and the deadly diseases that the infections can cause. Over the centuries humans were blaming god for anything they did not understand and were making up stories about gods intervention for punishment to warn the upcoming generations of the dangerous effects of such practices. Now that humans have a better understanding what dangerous infections can have on people and I think the more reasonable explanation is that those two cities were destroyed by the ravage effects of infections caused by the viruses and bacteria that are present in the stool of humans.

When humans do not learn from the history of past events, there is a possibility that history will repeat itself and the same thing will happen again on a global basis, only this time might wipe out the whole human race.

It is not reasonable to promote the so called pleasure of anal sexual activity, knowing very well the major risks and the ravage effects that can have on humans, this very controversial activity. If everyone start practicing anal sex for pleasure who is going to make the babies of the future generations. Anal sex alone produces no babies, and can cause sterility to men and women and other diseases making them unable to produce babies and that will affect the future of the human race and perhaps , and perhaps that will be the end of humans on this planet, like the dinosaurs !! The future will tell what will happen to humans from the controversial abnormal anal sexual activity .

These are some of the conditions caused by Unprotected receptive anal sex , HIV, human papillomavirus (HPV) (which can increase risk of anal cancer, typhoid fever, amoebas, Chlamydia, cryptosporidiosis, E. coli infections , giardiasis, gonorrhea, hepatitis A, B, And C, herpes simplex, Kaposi's sarcoma, (HHV-8) lymphogranuloma venereum, mycoplasma hominis , mycoplasma genital, pubic lice, salmonellas, shigella, syphilis, tuberculosis and other infections.

Now the million dollar question is: how can anyone, with a basic knowledge, that the feces comes out through the anus and has so many viruses and bacteria and the serious health risks that can cause, put his precious penis where all that dirt comes out? Is it worth the major risks for a few minutes of pleasure?   How can any intelligent person knowing all the health risks involved in this highly risky sexual activity, anal sex, allow anybody else to destroy their valuable anus   with such major risks? Perhaps people are either ignorant of the facts or are coerced and raped against their will. And that's is not   what consenting adults are doing in the privacy of their home , that is a non consenting sexual assault.

Over the centuries people had different sexual activities and among those activities was anal sex. Although there were laws in place against anal sex to protect the people from the ravaging effects of such an activity, many people in different countries they were breaking the law. Some of them were caught and punished for their acts but others   were practicing anal sex in secrecy.

In the last couple of centuries people practicing anal sex were organized and put pressure on governments to change the laws. In many countries the laws were abolished but in some countries they still have tough laws against anal sex to protect their citizens from abuse and the diseases that can cause such a practice. Time will prove who was right? those countries that abolished those laws or the countries that kept them for the protection of their citizens?

What is the normal natural

purpose of the sexual act?

The simple answer is , sex is for procreation and it was never intended for recreation or anything else. Sex is necessary for all living things to have offspring for the survival of their kind. Animals usually have sex just for procreation and almost never for recreation. From all the animal kingdom only man has created a whole sex industry for using and abusing their kind for profit. You will never find that in the rest of the animal kingdom. Humans exploited almost all parts of the human body for pleasure or profit. They use the usual sexual organs and unusual parts of the body, like the anus , the mouth, and other parts of the human body for personal gratification and many times for profit..

Lets examine each part of the body used for sex and see whether that's reasonable or not. What is the purpose of the female vagina in females? the vagina is part of the female sex organs and facilitates sexual activity for the purpose of the male penis to deposit the male sperms for the purpose of procreation. Vagina was created for normal sexual intercourse with the male sexual organ the penis. when the sperms are deposited in the vagina by the penis, the sperms swim towards the cervix the opening of the uterus, seeking the female egg to fertilize it and start a new baby. That is the main purpose of the sexual organs , to procreate a new life. In all the animal kingdom that's the purpose of the sexual act, that is to all except humans, which lost the purpose of sex and use sex for recreation using many parts of the human body for just pleasure.

ANATOMY AND PHYSIOLOGY OF THE FEMALE SEX ORGANS

The female primary sex organs are two, the ovaries which produce the female germ cells called OVARIES which they produce the female sex hormones ESTROGEN and progesterone. Estrogen and progesterone are responsible for the development of the female sex organs the vagina, uterus and the fallopian tubes and the mammary glands,(the two breasts of the females at puberty) . The female sex hormones ,Estrogen and progesterone are responsible for the development at puberty the appearance and maintenance of the secondary feminine characteristics of the females, development of breasts , pubic and auxiliary hair,

and female voice .
The ovaries produce the female eggs, once a month, which travel through the fallopian tubes towards the uterus seeking the male sperms for fertilization and the creation of a new baby.

The female sex organs' job is to facilitate the union of the female egg (ovum) with the incoming male sperm and after their union to form an embryo which will be attached to the uterus wall. With the successful attachment on the uterine wall the embryo will stay there getting its nourishment from the uterus via the placenta , grow to a new baby and when its fully grown and ready to come out to the world, it will do so and start a new life. So the female organs job is to facilitate the creation of a new life, a new baby. With the act of anal sexual activity , either voluntary on the part of the female or through coercion or force, the female organs are under the danger of loosing their normal function . The danger is that the female organs can have infections and sterility, causing those organs incapable to do what they were intended to do, the creation of a new life, a baby. And that will be a tragedy for the human race , leading to the demise of humans from the face of the earth.
So, for all the girls and women out there , if you want to be a mother and have babies someday , it

is sensible not to engage in highly risky sexual activities ,like the anal sex. If you are pressured by any male or female to have anal sex, send him/her packing. Because if you consent to anal sex, when your anus is not tight any more , he will damp you for another tight anus, and in the meantime you might loose your ability to have babies, or you can get other diseases too. Put yourself and your health first, and do not put your self at risk in order to please somebody's else abnormal desires. If he/she does not respect your wishes, he/she does not respect you as a person . All he is focused and concern is to please himself regardless if he can cause pain and harm to somebody else . I do not think you need such people in your life, but then again it is your body and your decision, nobody else can make decisions for you.

Here is a diagram of the female organs and their role in the sexual act.

1) the vagina which is used for the sexual act accommodating the male penis and receiving the spermatozoa. When the woman is still virgin, The opening of the vagina is covered with a thin layer of skin called hymen. The hymen's function is to keep germs and dirt out of vagina. that's why

women were supposed to be virgin until they get married, to make sure that their sexual organs were healthy and ready to produce babies.

2) the uterus, where the future embryo will attached itself and stay there for about nine months until it is time to come out and start a new life.
3) the two ovaries which produce the female eggs called ovum and
4) the two fallopian tubes which carry the ovum from the ovary to the uterus for fertilization.
When fertilization occurs the ovum which has the future baby is attached on the uterus wall to get the nutritional needs for the future baby from the mother's body through the placenta.
That is the purpose of the female organs, to facilitate the creation of the new baby. The female organs were never intended for recreation but only for procreation. when the female organs are sexually used and abused there is a possibility of infections and loose that ability to produce babies. That is called sterility.
Sometimes this process becomes impossible due to infections and blockage of the fallopian tubes. The egg from the ovaries cannot travel to the uterus for fertilization, thus the woman is unable to produce babies and becomes sterile. No human egg available for fertilization equals no possibility for any baby. The most common infections that

cause this blockage are due to sexually transmitted diseases , and germs from anal sex.

If women want to become mothers someday , and have children, it is wise to avoid any risky sexual activities. Protect your sexual organs from any risky sexual activity for a fleetly and questionable pleasure, and cherish your ability to create a new life, a new baby!

Perhaps that's why in some countries the men wanted their future wives to be virgins. They wanted the women to be healthy , free of any infections, and be able to have healthy children for their family.

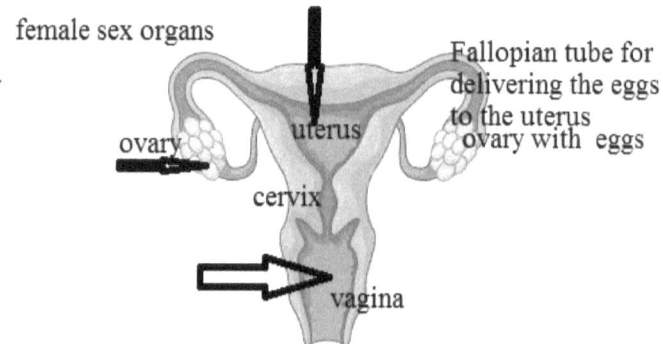

Unprotected anal sex followed by vaginal sex can transfer viruses and bacteria to the female sex organs which can cause blockage to the fallopian tubes making the woman sterile, because the female egg cannot travel from the ovary to the uterus to be fertilized by the spermatozoa. There are so many germs in the anus that can cause many infections and even cancer to the anus and the female organs. The risk is huge , so the women should be very careful if they want to have babies and become mothers some day.

One may think that men are always the perpetrator, and although that might be true, there are some exceptions, where women can be the perpetrator. During my research to write this book I saw in a book the picture of a female that she was abusing the anus of a man with a huge rubber penis attached to her pelvic area. I guess people will always find a way to hurt each other one way or the other. Using rubber sexual toys can do real damage to the human body and can transfer myriads of germs from contaminations. People abuse their bodies every day with abnormal activities and obnoxious substances all in the name of pleasure. As long as it is their bodies they are abusing or it is an activity between consenting adults and is not something illegal, it is their business . When their body pays the price they will have nobody else to blame but themselves.

Anyway, according to the laws of nature , a normal sexual activity is between a man and a woman with their normal sexual organs, penis to vagina intercourse to produce the future generation of humans. Anything else is out of   the normal sexual activity.

PURPOSE OF THE   MALE SEXUAL ORGANS

The male sex organs are two testicles which they produce the spermatozoa and the male sex hormone testosterone. The testosterone is responsible for the development of the secondary sex organs ,the penis, prostate gland, the epididymis (two), the vas deferens (two) ,seminal vesicles (two). And the secondary sex characteristics, deep voice due to laryngeal changes, pubic, facial and auxiliary hair.

The Male sex organs are located inside and outside the human body around the pubic bones.
1) the penis, a cylindrical organ made exactly to fit the vagina opening. The penis job is to transfer the spermatozoa to the female vagina during the normal vagina-penis sexual activity .
2) the scrotum is located at the base of the penis. The scrotum's job is to hold and support the human testicles.
3) two testicles that have egg like shape and are supported by the scrotum's sac . The testicle's job is to produce spermatozoa, the so called spermatogenesis, which starts after puberty and continues until old age. The spermatozoa when combine with the female egg will produce new babies. In other words the spermatozoa are the seeds of humans and when the have fertile ground, the female egg, produce a new life, a new baby.
4) the VAS DEFERENS , two small muscular tubes that contract and propel the spermatozoa

from the testicles to the penis' urethra.

5)two seminal vesicles which produce a viscous secretion to keep the spermatozoa alive and mobile.

6) the prostate gland and bulb urethral glands which produce a thin lubricant secretion.

During the sexual act the spermatozoa travel from the two testicles through the two vas deferens , the two seminal vesicles add more viscous fluid and from there passes through the urethra of the penis to deposit the seminal fluid containing several millions of spermatozoa in the female vagina. From there the spermatozoa race up through the vagina to the cervix of the uterus looking for the female egg to fertilize it and create a new baby. Out of the millions of spermatozoa that were deposited in the vagina by the male penis, only one or two spermatozoa will be able to fertilize the female egg and produce a baby.. that's the natural purpose of the sexual act.

For some reason the humans forgot that the sexual activity is for procreation and not for recreation.

WHAT IS THE NORMAL NATURAL FUNCTION OF THE ANUS?

Is it part of the sexual organs? of course NOT.

The anus is part of the long alimentary canal which starts from the mouth and ends at the anus. The purpose of the anus is for controlling and expelling the feces, the end waste byproduct of digestion. For this reason nature has provided the anus with strong circular muscles, the so called sphincters, to control the expulsion of the feces and avoid any accidental discharge. That is the real purpose of the anus and was never intended for anything else, and certainly never for sex. When the anus is used for sexual activity gradually the anal sphincter loose their function and gradually is unable to function properly and cannot control the feces causing fecal incontinence. In other words the anus cannot control the expulsion of the feces and accidents happen . People with that unfortunate predicament they have to use pampers. And

that's not the only side effect when abusing the anus for sexual activity.

The pros and cons of anal sex.

The pros of anal sex, if any.

Well, we very often hear from the proponents of anal sex the argument that anal sex is pleasurable. They talk about sexual pleasure because the anus is tight . Pleasure and more pleasure for the perpetrator, but how pleasurable is it to their victims, the ones that their anus is sexually abused? In an interview by a reporter of a man who was the victim of such abuse, he was talking about " painful as hell ", and not about pleasure.
Here are some of the pros for anal sex I found in the internet.
1) that you cannot get pregnant , which is true, but what about the myriad of health risks.
2) that it is a pleasurable activity.
Yes it might be Pleasurable to some and painful to others and with so many viruses and bacteria to cause havoc in your health………. Is it worth the risk?
3) they are talking that the sperm is nutritious and good for many conditions………. If that is the case, you can go to your butcher and order some animal testicles which are indeed very nutritious protein for your health without any health

risks……….zero risk.

4) that the anus is tight and provide pleasure during the anal sex…. Not a good excuse to cause injury and destruction of the anal sphincters, causing fecal incontinence and so many other risks……

However, tight was the vagina of the virgin girls too, but with repeated sex and with a childbirth or more it becomes loose and not so tight any more. The same thing happens to the anus too, with repeated anal sexual activity it will become loose and the owner of that anus will have problems holding the feces, causing fecal incontinence . And that is not the only risk for the person with an abused anus. The health risk are numerous and real, for the abused people. But The perpetrators will seek a new tight anus for their pleasure as soon as that abused anus is not tight anymore. There was a case in the paper sometimes ago, where a young man was sexually abused by the local church pastor and got HIV infection. In one of his interviews the young man was Saying that he thought that the pastor really loved him and that he and the pastor would always be together .But in one of their homosexual parties they had, the pastor got another young man for his sexual needs and passed him to another perpetrator for anal sexual abuse. The perpetrators groom their victims with empty promises but they rarely care for their victims .All they care about is about their pleasure that a tight anus will give them and it does not matter if it is a boy or a girl. As soon as their anus is not tight enough for their pleasure they look for another tight anus.

In another case, a female reporter from a local television station ,was interviewing a man who was sexually abused when he was growing up and at one time he had problems with his family and he went to live with his abuser for some time. At the time of the interview, this young man was strongly against this abnormal anal sexual practice and he was giving lectures against any anal sexual activity. He described how he was groomed and abused and he said ; " anal sex was painful like hell.' and then you have the perpetrators and proponents of anal sex to promote anal sex as a pleasurable activity. Perhaps to them it is a pleasurable activity but not to their victims.

Over the years I read in the papers and watched on television many cases of such abuses of innocent people , mainly children and youngsters of both sexes. All of them described their experience as painful and none of them as pleasurable.

But the advocates of anal sex are always pitching their own mantra, pleasure and more pleasure and nothing else. of course it is about their own pleasure they are talking about…

Besides similar pitches and promotions were used by the tobacco companies decades ago about their products. They were promoting their cigarettes as a glamorous pleasurable activity, and they use, actors, male and females to smoke their cigarettes in movies, videos and big advertising campaigns. The cigarettes companies as many other companies want to have people hooked on their products so that they have addicted slaves to use their products to make their profit. Exactly the same sales pitch the promoters of anal sex do, pleasure and more pleasure.

Now, a lot of innocent people are dying from cancer ,the side effects of smoking the cigarettes of the tobacco companies . The glamorous pleasure they were promised by the big tobacco companies is nowhere to be seen. And that's exactly what the perpetrators and promoters of anal sex are promising. Pleasure and more glamorous pleasure for them of course, and their victims will suffer the side effects and suffering of such an activity. Whatever consenting adults are doing in the privacy of their homes it is their own business and nobody's else, but do not glamorize anal sex as pleasurable activity. The health risks and side effect of the anal sexual abuse are too numerous and according to many anal abused people too painful to be considered as a pleasurable activity .

The cons of anal sexual activity.

There are so many health risks in engaging in this
abnormal sexual activity that one wonders why
take such risk for   merely a questionable pleasure.
Lets see what these health risks are and see if
there is any excuse that any logical   thinking
person can risk their health for merely a
questionable sexual pleasure.
The anus was never intended for any sexual
activity, therefore it lacks the natural lubrication
the vagina has. Any penetration of the anus can tear
the tissue inside the anus, allowing bacteria and
viruses that are present to enter the bloodstream
and cause severe infections. **The anus is full of
bacteria from the feces that is expelled by the
anus.** Even if both partners do not have a sexually-
transmitted infection or disease, bacteria normally
in the anus can potentially infect the giving partner
and the receiving partner. The tissue inside the anus
does not have this natural protection, which leaves
it vulnerable to tearing and the spread of infection.
The wall of the anus and rectum can be injured or
even perforated   which can be life threatening if
left untreated. It is extremely dangerous to insert
any sex toys in the anus which can cause severe
damage to the anus and rectum ,even life

threatening conditions. The giving partner can have urinary and other infections that can cause sterility and other diseases.

Due to the many viruses and bacteria present in the fecal matter that passes through the anal canal here are some of the infections that can cause during anal sex. Studies have suggested that anal exposure to HIV poses 30 times more risk for the receptive partner than vaginal exposure. Exposure to the human papillomavirus (HPV) may also lead to the development of anal warts and anal cancer. **Other infections include anal herpes, anal warts, anal abscesses, anal fissures, parasites and a lot more infections depending of what bacteria and viruses are available in the fecal matter that passes through the anus.**

The anus was designed to hold the waste products of digestion , also known as feces and repetitive anal sex may lead to weakening of the anal sphincter, making it difficult to hold in feces until you can get to the toilet and that is called fecal incontinence. Many people practicing anal sex end up using pads and pampers for protection from any accidental fecal discharge.

Anal sex is the riskiest form of any sexual activity and anyone can wonder why take such risks for merely some fleeting pleasure. Anal sex can cause urinary tract infections and even sterility to both men and women.

Rao Camini in his book " principles and practice of assisted reproductive technology" writes; "Unprotected anal sex is a risk factor for formation of antisperm antibodies (ASA) in the recipient. In some people, ASA may cause autoimmune infertility.[90] Antisperm antibodies impair fertilization, negatively affect the implantation process and impair growth and development of the embryo.[91][90] """

Comparing the Sexual habits of humans to other animals.

In the animal kingdom , sex is simple. They have sex for procreation and never for recreation. If you ever lived in a farm and you had animals , you know that the animals have the so called breeding or mating season. The animals instinctively know that it is time to mate , have sexual activity for the purpose of producing the new generation of their kind. The male animals have a job to do, to impregnate the female animal and produce babies.

Sometimes they have to fight other male animal in the same herd to have the exclusive rights of that job with the female animals. Their fight last until there is a winner, the stronger male will have the right to impregnate the females with his spermatozoa and make strong healthy babies.

Humans are completely different. They lost the sense of the mating season. They have sex at any time for recreation and sometimes they are not interested in procreation but just for pleasure. They have sex just for pleasure and they created big profitable industries out of the sexual activity. There is no comparison of the animal sexual activity and the human sexual activity. The animals have the right idea about sex , for procreation and the humans are lost and the only thing they are interested , is pleasure and more pleasure . In their pursuit of pleasure, they use and sexually abuse almost every part of their bodies. Humans have no boundaries of their sexual pleasures. Sometimes they use and abuse the females as their slaves. I was watching jerry Springer, the host of "The **Jerry Springer** Show" in one of his shows where a man brought his girlfriend with a leash on her neck introducing her as his sex slave. There are a lot of people that for some reason agree, or forced to such a situation, and trained to please their partners or masters as they called them.   And people thought that slavery was a thing of the past.

I think that animals behavior towards sex is a lot better than the human behavior. The animals follow the natures way for procreation and the humans choose the recreational way, pleasure and more pleasure , no matter if they hurt other human beings.

Another dangerous human sexual practice is the Oral sex?

The oral cavity, commonly known as the mouth was meant for the feeding the body for its nutritional needs. That's why people eat their daily food for the body's fuel needs. How this cavity was involved in the sexual activity is a mystery. In ancient Roman texts they used oral sex , also known as fellatio, as a punishment for petty thefts and other minor crimes. Anyway, I guess humans will always think of some excuse to use any part of the body for their sexual gratifications.

Oral sexual activity is as dangerous as anal sex. Participants in oral sex can get many sexual transmitted diseases and then some . Participants in such sexual activity can have oral cancer from the same virus that causes cancer in the sexual organs,, human papilloma virus (HPV) (which can increase risk of anal cancer,)

People in different parts of the world have different excuses in practicing oral sex. Women practicing oral sex on men can have testosterone side effects, like growing facial hair and changing their voice like a male's voice.

THE PURPOSE OF THE SEXUAL ACTIVITY FOR ALL LIVING CREATURES.

In simple words, the purpose of sex in all creatures is for procreation and it was never intended for recreation. Most of the animals they know when the female is ready for procreation and they engage in sexual activity to accomplish that task. When I was young, living in a farm, there were many farm animals that they were doing exactly that. We could see the male sheep ram sniffing the air to see which female sheep was ovulating and was ready for procreation. After a few minutes it was zeroing in on the sheep that was sending the signals that she was ready. The ram was rushing to her smelling her vagina and proceeding to do his duty delivering his spermatozoa to the waiting female egg for fertilization. Once he finished his duty with that female sheep he would sniff the air again to see which other female sheep was needing his assistance to procreate. He was doing that every day until all mature female sheep were impregnated and then he would stop sniffing the air. He never bother any immature females that were not ready for procreation. The rest of the year he would eat, drink and be happy until the next breeding season.

This ritual is happening in all animals. Their sexual activity is mainly for procreation with mature ovulating females of their kind. They usually have a breeding season when they are sexually active and the rest of the time they just live normal lives without any sexual interest or sexual activity. The animals are living their sexual lives for the purpose that sex was intended, procreation for reproduction and multiplication of their kind. Humans fulfill that need for procreation and reproduction but that is not the only purpose of their sexual activity. Humans have created a huge sex industry of billions of dollars with the only purpose for recreation. Humans have lost their way about the true purpose of sex.

They try to satisfy their sexual needs for the purpose of pleasure and more pleasure. In their desire to achieve as much pleasure as possible they exploited   all parts of the human body and then some. They created many sex toys to use and enhance their pleasure. Some of those sex toys are dangerous and can harm people, but that does not stop them. They use and abuse the young and vulnerable , all in the name of pleasure and profit. Many humans are only interested in sexual recreation and they pursue their dream for more sexual pleasure by destroying the lives of many young and vulnerable people. There is no limit to their sexual appetite for pleasure.

Any laws that were put there to protect the young and the innocent are constantly challenged and abolished , leaving the young and vulnerable defenseless to their abnormal sexual desires.

Animals live by the laws of nature but humans live by the laws of pleasure and more pleasure,   which they can change any law according to their sexual desire and preferences   of the season and who can outwit the rest of the humans with their politics and rhetoric.

Where all this destructive path will lead the humans , it is anybody's guess. But with all the infections and diseases that this human trend brings, it is possible that humans might end up with the same fate as Sodom and Gomorrah had. Time will tell.

POTENTIAL HEALTH RISKS TO

BOTH PARTIES OF ANAL SEX

Anal sex used to be practiced only by men but nowadays anal sex is practiced by both men and women. It is the latest fad of modern times spreading in all socioeconomic levels of society. Every time people engage in anal sexual activity, consciously or unconsciously , they put their health in danger due to the fact that the anus is full of pathogenic germs that can cause serious infections even life threatening diseases . No matter what precautions they take there is always a risk of infections due to the fact that out of the anus comes the end byproduct of digestion, called feces . Fecal contamination of anything is a serious health risk to humans. That's why nature gave the feces the offensive smell and the myriad of germs to dissuade humans from any sexual inappropriate action there. However, humans ignore all the nature's warnings and they have anal sex, seeking a fleetly pleasure. Nature has a way to punish those that disrespect the nature's laws.

Here are some of the nature's punishments to those that disrespect the normal sexual activity and engage in the unnatural anal sexual activity.

For men and women engaging in anal sexual activity these are some of the serious health risks.

Anal incontinence , rectal perforation , anal injuries with bleeding and infections, bladder and kidney infections, sterility dew to infections for both parties, cancer and many other diseases. In women that practice anal sex there is a risk of cancer, infections to bladder and kidneys, infections and blockage to the fallopian tubes causing sterility and other conditions.

For any woman or man that want to have children some day, they should think it seriously before embarking in such a highly risky sexual activity that might cause them to be sterile and unable to have children.

THE ROLE OF CHURCH IN ANAL SEXUAL ACTIVITY   OVER THE YEARS.
THE CHURCH CLERGY HAVE BEEN PREYING ON THE YOUNG for many years with immunity!

For years the church   hierarchy was preaching that anal sex was a blasphemy and against the god's will and against the church's policy. The church even was talking about other sexual activities   between consenting heterosexual activities as sins and against the gods will.

However over the years the church people were preaching one thing and practicing something else, with millions of male and females youngsters sexually abused by the priests. A simple search in the internet will provide many examples of sexual abuse by the pastors…………Here are a few below..

[[**20 years, 700 victims: Southern Baptist sexual abuse spreads as ...**

https://www.houstonchronicle.com/.../Southern-Baptist-sexual-abuse-spreads-as-leader...

Feb 10, 2019 - This collection of mug shots includes a portion of the 220 *people* who, since 1998, ... In 2007, victims of *sexual abuse* by Southern Baptist *pastors* ... Two *other* former *members* of the man's *churches* said in interviews that they ...

'men of God' sexually abused children. Then they found refuge at other ...
https://www.star-telegram.com/living/religion/article222576430.html
Dec 9, 2018 - A pattern of cover-ups and the shuffling of suspected abusers among *churches* and universities that are part of the independent fundamental ...

The Privilege of Predators: Church Sexual Abuse And Society's ...
https://centerforinquiry.org/blog/the-privilege-of-predators/

Aug 15, 2018 - A new Grand Jury report details the overwhelming *sexual abuse* by over 300 Pennsylvania ... But priests, we are told, are good *people*. ... by the Catholic Church

at various levels of its *hierarchy*, the abuse is an ongoing crisis. ... *Other* Christian *denominations*, such as the Jehovah's Witnesses, Mormons, …]]

There were sexual abuses by the church people all over the world and that's the tip of the iceberg.
I am sure there are sexual abuses in other religions as well .

Child sexual abuse inquiry to be held into religious organisations ...

https://www.theguardian.com/.../child-sexual-abuse-inquiry-to-be-held-religious-organis...

3 days ago - Investigation will include *Christian*, Islamic, Jewish and Buddhist organizations. ... Child *sexual abuse* in a wide range of *religious* organizations and settings, ... schools, will be investigated, along with *faith*-based *youth* groups and camps. ... of child *sexual abuse* and *other* mistreatment in Jehovah's Witness ...

THE PEDOPHILES ARE PREYING ON THE YOUNG.

There are pedophiles everywhere preying on the young, sexually abusing boys and girls of all ages. You can find these people in almost all organizations . You can find reporting of these abuses in the media, and that's only the tip of the iceberg. Only the ones that were caught and brought to justice are reported, but there are many other sexually abused people that did not report their abuse. The abused, are either afraid of their abuser, or they think that it is their fault and feel guilty. When one of the abused decides to come forward and report the abuser , other abused come out and tell their

stories. Like the story with the doctor abusing the U.S.A. Olympic athletes for years. And many other cases too many to write about. A search in the internet about these abuses will shock you. Here are a few .
[[
Britain shocked by growing soccer child abuse scandal | CBC Sports
https://www.cbc.ca/sports/soccer/britain-soccer-sexual-abuse-children-1.3876322

Dec 1, 2016 - The allegations of child *sex abuse* in English soccer from the 1970s ... lifted the lid on what could be one of the worst *pedophile* scandals Britain has ... BBC television star who abused hundreds of *youngsters* over six decades.

French child rape case is another lesson about sports abuse ...
www.startribune.com/french-child-rape-case-is-another...sports-abuse/504792232/

Jan 24, 2019 - French child rape case is another lesson about *sports* abuse ... raping and *sexually assaulting* children, was that the ex-elite athlete — like other notorious *sports* officials and coaches — was using his position to brutalize *young people*. ... how to combat *pedophilia in sports* and sharing his experience as a ...]]]

All the pedophiles have one thing in common. They are interest for their own pleasure and more pleasure, sexually abusing their victims and do not care if they ruin the lives of their victims. I watched a female reporter interviewing and pedophile who spend many years in prison for his sexually abusing children and he was admitting that all he always wanted is to abuse kids for his own pleasure and nothing else. these people tend to offend and re-offend again and again and it is the menace of kids and society with no chance of rehabilitation. Television and other media regularly report such cases.

SEX EDUCATION 101

Sex education at home

Sex education should start at home by the parents. It is the parents responsibility to teach their kids about sex and their life values. The parents should teach their kids from an early age about their private parts with the normal names of each sexual organ. They should also teach them that their private sex organs are private and that nobody else should tough them there. If anybody tries to touch their privates, they should report it to their parents right away. Of course they should tell them that the kids should never touch the private parts of other kids or grown ups.

They should also teach the kids that their anus is the part of the digestive system, and its function is to expel the byproducts of digestion called feces. They should also teach them that anything that comes out of the anus is dirty and full germs, which can cause infections. The food that goes through the mouth for the nutritional needs of the body and finally after the process of digestion ends up at the anus to be expelled. The gastrointestinal tract which starts from the mouth where people eat their food and after a long journey through the gastrointestinal tract, the body absorbs what it needs and the rest is expelled through the anus as the waste byproduct of digestion. Anything that comes out of the anus is dirty and full of germs and has a foul smell to warn people that it is dangerous to health. Every time they have to go to the washroom they should wash their hands to avoid any germs that cause infections. Good hygiene is essential for good health.

They should also teach their kids why boys and girls sexual organs are different and be proud of what they got, it is a priceless gift from nature. Nature provides the girls with their sex organs and the boys with their sex organs and when the grow up they will be able to have babies of their own. They should teach boys that their sexual organs,   when they grow up and are mature enough will produce the spermatozoa , In other words the seeds that when combined with the mature eggs of the women will produce their babies.

They should teach the girls that although nature did not give them a penis, nature gave them the greatest gift of all, the ability to make babies. Teach them that their sexual organs are different than the boys but they have the ability to produce eggs and when the eggs combine with sperm of boys when they grow up they will procreate a new life, new babies.

They should also teach the kids that in order to be able to have their own kids someday, they should take good care of themselves and not experiment with any sexual activity until they are mature and ready to face the responsibilities of having babies.

Parents should answer any questions that their kids might ask, with clarity and honesty.

The parents should warned their kids about the sexual predators and tell them to avoid talking to strangers and that even friends of the family should not engage with them in any physical contact involving their private parts.

<u>Parents should be on the look out for possible child molesters and predators among their friend, neighbors and relatives.</u> Many kids are sexually abused by family friends, neighbors

and relatives. There was a woman on the DR. Oz who was telling her story , how she, her sister and mother were molested and sexually abused for years by the best friend of her father. He even manage to manipulate her father to sexually relieve him with masturbating him in his cars. Sometimes I wonder how gullible and trusty people can be ! But it can happen. The parents responsibility is to protect their kids and not to worry if they will offend the deviant behavior of their friends or relatives.

They should also warn them about the dangers of the internet and they should never chat with strangers in chat rooms and never send any pictures of themselves nude or with clothes because you never know where those pictures will end up…
They should also tell them about bullying and that they can come to them with for help with any questions or concerns they might have.
Kids need to know that their parents are their to protect them from any danger or threat. Encourage them to ask any question they might have…….

Where do the babies come from?
If they ask where do the babies come from, just tell them the truth; from their mothers womb

and explain to them that women have the exclusive privilege to make babies and that the men have the privilege to produce the seeds that enable women to have babies.

How are babies made? A seed from the daddy and an egg from the mommy join together to create a new baby in the mommy's tummy. That's how the baby is made and it grows in a special sack in the mother's womb until it is ready to come out and start a new life.

The parents should always answer any question their kids ask them. That is the only way to teach your kids the values you want them to have.

Sex education in schools

The school sex education should be done separate for boys and girls so that kids are not embarrassed to ask questions. Although the sex education is done separately for boys and girls, they should teach both boys and girls about the anatomy and physiology of both sexes.

They should teach the kids about the role the males and females have in the procreation process. The gifts they have from nature as males and females. They should emphasize that any sexual act has its consequences and that they should not rush into anything before they grow up and are mature enough to take care of their responsibilities. Sex is a serious matter with serious consequences. Any sexual activity can   be dangerous to their health from the sexual transmitted diseases.

They should teach them that if they want to be mothers or fathers someday ,that they have to be very careful about their sex life . With any sexual activity there is a risk   of serious infections which can cause serious diseases including cancer and sterility.

Sex is not always about fun and pleasure, sex is a serious business

  with serious consequences, like pregnancy to the females, and potential serious health risks to every one engaging in any sexual activity .

School sex education should teach the kids the truth about sex , anal sex , vagina sex and any other type of sex and never ever bend the truth to satisfy any new FAD or   the few that always seek a tight anus for pleasure at the expense of others. The schools should teach the kids the truth that the anus is not part of the sexual organs and it was never indented for any sexual activity. They should teach the kids that   anal sex is very dangerous to their   health because of the many germs and viruses that are present there from the feces that comes out from the anus. The schools should never bend the truth   about anal sex, trying to be politically correct because of nay new fad on the horizon and some people like to practice anal sex for their recreation.

If some people like to practice anal sex that does not mean that anal sex is not without potential health risks, no matter who likes to do that.

The schools should tell the kids the truth about the dangers associated with any sexual activity and especially any sexual anal activity.

Whatever consenting adults are doing in the privacy of their homes, or the choices they make, it is their own business and nobody's else, but the schools cannot bend the truth or lie to the kids because some people ignore the risks and practice risky sexual activities . The kids and everybody else should be taught the truth about the risky anal sexual activity and if knowing the risks associated with such an activity, choose to have such a risky activity, it is up to them and nobody else. When their health pays the price, at least they cannot blame anybody else for the choice they made.

Anal sex is a highly risky sexual activity no matter who does it, even if he is the most powerful man or woman on earth. As a matter of fact any sexual activity is a risky activity but the anal sex is more dangerous because of what comes out of the anus, the feces, which always has harmful bacteria and viruses that can cause serious life threatening diseases. The school kids should learn that in school. Teach the kids the truth and nothing but the truth, that's what education means.

A good sexual education at home by answering all the questions to the kids and a good education about sex at school, will arm the kids with the knowledge needed to make the right decisions about their sexual activities and their choices in life.

The distinction between love and sex

People usually confuse the sexual act as making love, which is definitely not correct. Sex is a physical act and anyone can do without any love. Animals do it all the time without any feeling of love, just the sexual act for procreation. that's what the sexual act is a physical act. Some people even try to have sex with someone by telling them " if you love me, you will have sex with me''. this is a cheap excuse to pressure someone, mostly women to have sex with their boyfriends. Some women fall for this pressure and they have sex with them, but other women have a good answer to that.

"If you really love me, you will respect my wishes and you will not pressure me to do something that I am not comfortable with and I am not ready to do yet". that is the perfect answer to an unwanted pressure to have sex with someone you do not want to be intimate with .

Love on the other hand is a feeling that comes within and there are different types of love according to the situation. You have a love for your parents, love for your siblings, love for your friends, love for your job, love for your country and of course love for your lover. Each type of love is different than that of your lover and even that one some times does not last for ever. However the feeling of loving someone , or to be loved by someone is a wonderful feeling and if that last for ever you are a very lucky person indeed. That is a feeling that sex alone will never replace, as sex is more of a physical desire that can fade fast. And then you have unconditional love of a mother which lasts forever.

There are five camps in the anal sex saga .

1) in the first place are the perpetrators , the advocates and proponents of anal sex the so call, Anusphile (one that is obsessed with having anal sex) . These guys always like a tight anus of someone's else but never if ever let anyone to penetrate their anus. As soon as that anus becomes too loose for their taste they look for a new tight anus to wreck with their penis or toys. Most of these guys are serial pedophiles and they seek to have sex with children both male and females. They do not even call themselves homosexuals, or gays but they can be classified as bisexual. Over the years I heard many such cases on television, newspapers and radio. In one such case two

ushers in a hockey arena they used to let kids in the arena to watch the hockey games for free with the condition of anal with the kids in exchange. This went on for a long time and many kids were sexually abused by the two ushers. The victims of the two ushers never said anything about their abuse because either they were ashamed or they thought that the ushers were doing them a favor and the sexual abuse was a way to repay them for letting them watch the hockey games for free. There are many, many such cases that I read on newspapers or television and I could write many books of thousands of pages.

Guys like These two guys are the most vocal and proponents of anal sex. They want to protect and promote their practice so that they continue their sexual practice without any legal punishment. You can find these sexual predators in all socioeconomic levels of society and in all jobs and professions. They often use their position and influence to affect the laws and attitude of society.

The newspapers and televisions report their sexual scandals very often. A recent such a predatory scandal was that of the catholic's church scandal in which thousands of kids were abused by the churches' representatives. It seems that young boys and girls are sexually abused by those that they were supposed to protect them, teachers, policemen, lawyers, politicians, clergymen and rare occasions even their own parents or ralatives.

These are the perpetrators that seek every opportunity to change the existing laws that protect the young and the vulnerable so that they can protect their own turf and practice their   devious anal sexual   preference with immunity.

 Here are some of the reports of such abuse in the internet.

*https://www.dw.com/en/polands-catholic-**church**-admits-**clergy**...*

*News Poland's Catholic **Church** admits **clergy sexually abused** hundreds of **children**. Poland's Catholic **Church** has released a report admitting hundreds of clergymen **abused children** ...*

*https://www.smalljoys.tv/illinois-priests-**abusing-children***

*Illinois Attorney General has issued a damning report about **clergy sexual abuse** on Wednesday, saying that the names of more than 500 **clergy** accused of **sexually abusing children** haven't yet released by the state's Catholic dioceses.*

 You can find   many such reports about clergy and others in authority....

One can only wonder where the society is heading?

2) In the second place are the victims of the above perpetrators . They were groomed and brainwashed by their abusers and they made them believe that their sexual anal abuse is something that they sought after. Their abusers established a predatory relationship and they have their victims under their control for their sexual abuse. The people in this category, who in reality are the victims are either ashamed or they accept their fate in the situation they are in. They rarely complain or report their abusers to authorities because they feel ashamed or have good report with their abusers or they think that it was their fault and nobody will listen to them. Only god knows how many million of people are sexually abused every year and they never report it to anyone. Some of them are even calling themselves gays or homosexuals and they want to be left alone with their predicament. One of the many abused kids by the ushers in the hockey arena mentioned above, finally had the courage to speak out and spilled the beans of what was happening in that place. By then he was in his mid -twenties and engaged to a girl his own age. He went to the local newspaper and described with all the sordid details how he and the other kids were groomed and abused by the two ushers. The ushers were dining and entertaining the kids organizing sexual parties where they were sexually abused and encouraging the kids to have sexual acts among the kids. The ushers made the kids believe that they were homosexuals and had that belief for many years. After telling his story to the local paper the police was involved and investigated his story. After a prolong investigation the police finally charged the two ushers for sexually abusing him and   they went to prison for some time. Unfortunately for the young lad he had many psychological problems from his sexual abuse that he put an end to his life. Even though it was never his fault for his sexual abuse he was feeling guilty and remorse for allowing himself to be sexually abused and many   abused kids feel the same way.

 It is unfortunate but that's how a lot of abused kids grow up thinking this way and live their lives feeling ashamed of the predicament they are in.

  Society   should teach the young kids that whenever they are sexually abused it is never the kids fault and   they should report the abuse immediately so that the perpetrators are recognized and stopped early . Even when they grow up and they are mature adults should speak up and name their abuser and sue them for their abuse. That is the only way to stop the abusers from abusing other kids. The "me too movement" which started with the abused women naming their abusers and taking them to courts , is a good start . All the abused people, male and females should speak up and name their abusers to stop this sexual abuse.

Abused people develop physical and psychological problems and Some of these abused kids go on to become sexual perpetrators and abuse other innocent kids .

3) In the third place are the gullible people, you can even buy the snake oil from a snake salesman. These are the people that either they do not care or easily persuaded and accept any new fad or trend. These people are easily dubbed , manipulated and easily abused. They will believe anybody of what they tell them. They can easily be persuaded to support and participate in any normal or abnormal activity. You can find them in any socioeconomic level of every society.

4) in the fourth place are people concerned about the results of such a practice will have on society and the future of the human race. These are the people that are concerned about the health of their children. They worry that such activity will ruin the future of their kids and society as a whole. With horror they watch one law after the other crumpled and abolished in favor of the loud demands of the few . The various advocates of such activities , their societies and their supporters are gaining ground everywhere and they manage to establish liaisons with the government and the schools and they teach school kids false information about the anal sex and that worries the people that their kids are in danger of abuse. Unfortunately , although these people are rightly concerned about such practices, they are loosing control of what their kids can and cannot learn in the school. We already see that due the false teachings in schools and the abolishing of protective laws, a lot of kids are facing sexual anal abuse by their peers .

Below is a study done in England and published in the BMJ . This study is published on the creative commons .

, " the study, published on BMJ Open, says Anal heterosexual among young people and implications for health promotion: a qualitative study in the UK

C Marston,
R Lewis

A study on why teenage heterosexual couples may engage in anal sex has revealed a climate of coercion, with consent and mutuality not always a priority for the boys who are trying to persuade girls into having it.

Researchers at the London School of Hygiene and Tropical Medicine interviewed 130 teenagers aged

16-18 in three sites across the country to "explore expectations, experiences and circumstances of anal sex among young people".

The qualitative study found that anal heterosexual appeared to be **"painful, risky and coercive, particularly for women",** while **males spoke of being expected to persuade or coerce reluctant partners.**

"Anal sex is increasingly prevalent among young people, yet anal intercourse between men and women—although commonly depicted in sexually explicit media—is usually absent from mainstream sexuality education and seems unmentionable in many social contexts," the study, published on *BMJ Open*, says.

It found that some **young people normalized "coercive, painful and unsafe anal sex",** in an issue that needs to be addressed by health workers and schools in sex education.

Sexually active people are engaging in anal sex more than ever before, the researchers said of other recent studies, and in this one, they usually **occurred between boys and girls within boyfriend/girlfriend relationships.**

The interviewed young people rarely spoke of anal sex "in terms of mutual exploration of sexual pleasure", while condoms were also often not used. There appeared to be competition between boys to have had anal sex with girls, while the main reason that young people also cited for engaging in the act is that boys **"wanted to copy what they saw in pornography and that 'it's tighter'"**.

The researchers also found examples of non-consensual penetration either with a finger or penis in a 'try it and see' approach in the hope the girl would not stop them.

The researchers also found examples of non-consensual penetration either with a finger or penis in a 'try it and see' approach in the hope the girl would not stop them.

"**Some events, particularly the 'accidental' penetration** reported by some interviewees, were ambiguous in terms of whether or not **they would be classed as rape (i.e., non-consensual penetration),** but we know from [one] interview that 'accidents' may happen on purpose," after a respondent admitted telling his girlfriend that he had accidentally penetrated her anally, **when in fact he had done it on purpose.**

Anal heterosexual among young people and implications for health promotion: a qualitative study in the UK
    C Marston,
    R Lewis
Author affiliations

Abstract

Objective To explore expectations, experiences and circumstances of anal sex among young people.

Design Qualitative, longitudinal study using individual and group interviews.

Participants 130 men and women aged 16–18 from diverse social backgrounds.

Setting 3 contrasting sites in England (London, a northern industrial city, rural southwest).

Results Anal heterosexual often appeared to be painful, risky and coercive, particularly for women. Interviewees frequently cited pornography as the 'explanation' for anal sex, yet their accounts revealed a complex context with availability of pornography being only one element. Other key elements included competition between men; the claim that 'people must like it if they do it' (made alongside the seemingly contradictory expectation that it will be painful for women); and, crucially, normalization of coercion and 'accidental' penetration. **It seemed that men were expected to persuade or coerce reluctant partners**.

Conclusions Young people's narratives normalized coercive, painful and unsafe anal heterosexual. This study suggests an urgent need for harm reduction efforts targeting anal sex to help encourage discussion about mutuality and consent, reduce risky and painful techniques and challenge views that normalize coercion.

As we see from the above article the youngsters are practicing more often   anal sex due to the false information they get from pornographic videos and perhaps from other sources and maybe even from the sex education in schools.   Male and females are in danger of anal Sexual abuse . Teenage boys used to have girlfriends for vaginal sex but now they want to abuse   the girls in any way they can and parents and society are rightly concerned about these developments. The future of the humans is in danger from the used and abuse of this abnormal anal sexual activity.

5)in the fifth place are those that they chose to have only homosexual sexual activity. These people call themselves , gays, homosexuals, lesbians etc. homosexuality is a sexual attraction or behavior between members of the same sex. Contrary to the common belief that all homosexuals have anal sex, that is not true according to several studies.

Besides what consenting adults choose to do in the privacy of their homes it is their own business no matter if they are homosexuals, heterosexuals, bisexuals or anything else.

However, no matter who is practicing anal sex, the fact is that anal sex , is dangerous to the people engaging in anal sexual activity with so many potential health risks. If people are aware of the many health risks of such activity and still go ahead and do it , it is a health risk that someday may live to regret it.

The purpose of this book is not to judge consenting adults what they do with their private lives, but just to emphasize that anal sex is the sexual abuse of a non sexual organ with potentially huge health risks, no matter who does it. It does not matter if they are heterosexual, bisexual men or women or anything else, the anal sexual activity is an abuse of a non sexual organ . It is a health risk that put the future of humans in danger. We cannot bent the truth because some people like to abuse their anuses or other people anuses.

Anal sex is an abuse of the anus and that is the truth according to the anatomy and physiology of the

human body and the laws of nature. As long as consenting adults do whatever they want to do in the privacy of their homes, it is their own business and nobody's else, no matter if their men or women. But that does not mean that is right or without any health concerns or consequences.
If people want to ignore the potential health risks of anal sex and go ahead and do it, it is their business. People abuse their bodies in many other ways, such as smoking, drinking drugs and other dangerous activities. People are free to make their own decisions about their own bodies and lifestyles.
In this book I sound the alarm of the myriad of potential health risks and if some people listen and stop having any anal sexual activity for their own health, that's good but if they don't, that's ok too. After all it is their body, their health and their decision.. If their health finally pays the price, they have nobody else to blame.

Below is a free newsletter that discusses many health issues by the Mayo clinic staff. You can find it in the internet with many other e-newsletters about many topics.

Health issues for gay men and men who have sex with men

Understand important health issues for gay men and men who have sex with men — from sexually transmitted infections to depression — and get tips for taking charge of your health.

By Mayo Clinic Staff

Many doctors and institutions that deal with the health issues arising from any anal sexual activity, raise the alarm about the impending health risks of such sexual activity. It is all in the internet , and all you have to do is to search the internet about the health risks of anal sex.

Here are some of their comments I found in the internet when I was searching for "medical opinion on anal sex"

1):://www.medicalnewstoday.com/articles/156549.php

Anal cancer is a tumor that grows in the anus or **anal** canal. It is a rare form of cancer that tends to be more common in women than men. Risk factors

include infection with the human papilloma ...
2)A rare, but serious, complication after anal sex is a hole (perforation) in the colon. This dangerous problem requires hospitalization, surgery to repair the hole, and antibiotics to prevent infection.
3)The research, published in the **medical** journal BMJ Open, attempted to collect information about when **anal sex** occurs and the reasons why men and women engage in it.
Author: Kristen Sollee   "'''''''''''''

There so many medical opinions warning against anal sex that one can write many books about it. Do your own internet research and see for your self if you are interested or have any doubts..

THE COURT DECISION THAT ABOLISHED THE LAW PROTECTING THE YOUNGSTERS from anal sex.

Here is the law that was protecting the people under 18 from anal sexual abuse. The law was clear when anal sex was permitted and when it was not, and you do not have to be a lawyer to understand it. It is written in plain English, but somehow the judges can interpret it anyway they like, if they mixed the laws with the constitution or the potential rights of the individual. Later on we will see how a single judge can repeal and abolish any law with their rulings

The law as it was written to protect youngsters from anal sex.

.

Anal intercourse
- **159** (1) Every person who engages in an act of anal intercourse is guilty of an indictable offence and liable to imprisonment for a term not exceeding ten years or is guilty of an offence punishable on summary conviction.
- Marginal note: Exception

(2) Subsection (1) does not apply to any act engaged in, in private, between

- (a) husband and wife, or
- (b) any two persons, each of whom is eighteen years of age or more,

both of whom consent to the act.

- Marginal note: Idem

(3) For the purposes of subsection (2),

- (a) an act shall be deemed not to have been engaged in in private if it is engaged in in a public place or if more than two persons take part or are present; and
- (b) a person shall be deemed not to consent to an act
  - (i) if the consent is extorted by force, threats or fear of bodily harm or is obtained by false and fraudulent misrepresentations respecting the nature and quality of the act, or
  - (ii) if the court is satisfied beyond a reasonable doubt that the person could not have consented to the act by reason of mental disability.

-
- R. S., 1985, c. 19 (3rd Supp.), s. 3.
-
- Take a look at the criminal code, it's right there, in Section 159.

"Every person who engages in an act of anal intercourse is guilty of an indictable offence and liable to imprisonment for a term not exceeding ten years or is guilty of an offence punishable on summary conviction," it reads.

If you're married and if both consenting partners are over

18 it is legal but if not, off to the slammer with you, bud. It's also illegal if "it is engaged in in a public place or if more than two persons take part or are present." So no anal three ways are allowed by the government of Canada.

For those of you keeping count, 18 is two years older than 16—the typical age of consent in Canada

But, fear not, because, according to the Huffington Post, at the start of next week the Liberal government are expected to bring forward legislation on Tuesday that would repeal Section 159.

Here is how a single judge repealed and abolished the above law.

This is the case that was before the courts and the judge made that historic decision.

The details are described below in the court decision , but here is a short description of what happened. A man was charged for having sex including anal sex with the niece of his fiancé which started when she was 13 and he was 23. Anybody that reads the criminal code section 159 , should expect that he would be found guilty for having sex with a minor. However the judge found him not guilty and he was acquitted and the Crown appealed that decision.

During the second trial , the judge not only

acquitted that man for having all sorts of sexual activity including anal sex with that underage girl , but went a step further by abolishing the law that was there to protect youngsters under 18. The judge's reasoning , well read that decision below. Was the judge right or wrong for that decision? You make your own judgment.

Here is the full details of the case as it was reported in the court's ruling.

Regina v. Carmen M.
[Indexed as: R. v. M. (C.)]
23 O.R. (3d) 629
[1995] O.J. No. 1432
No. C12929
Court of Appeal for Ontario
Goodman, Catzman and Abella JJ.A.
May 24, 1995
Charter of Rights and Freedoms -- Equality rights -- Discrimination on basis of age -- Section 159 of Criminal Code (prohibiting anal intercourse unless both consenting individuals are at least 18 years old or married) discriminatory on basis of age contrary to s. 15(1) of Charter -- Discriminatory effect of s. 159 not justified under s. 1 of Charter -- Section 159 of no force or effect -- Canadian Charter of Rights and Freedoms, ss. 1, 15(1) -- Criminal Code, R.S.C. 1985, c. C-46, s. 159.
The accused was charged with a number of offences, including anal intercourse contrary to s. 159 of the Criminal Code, arising out of a three-year affair with the

niece of his fiancée which started when the complainant was 13 and the accused was 23. The trial judge found that the acts of anal intercourse took place when the complainant was between 14 and 18 years old, and that she had consented to them. She found that s. 159 of the Code, which prohibits anal intercourse unless both parties consent and are at least 18 years old or married, violated s. 7 of the Canadian Charter of Rights and Freedoms because it deprived an accused of the defense of consent. She therefore read this defense into s. 159, concluded that the accused was entitled to avail himself of the defense, and found him not guilty of anal intercourse. The Crown appealed.

Held, the appeal should be dismissed.

Per Abella J. A.: Anyone who is 14 or older, whether married or not, can consent to most forms of non-exploitive sexual conduct without criminal consequences, whereas no one can consent to anal intercourse unless he or she is at least 18 or married. Sexual orientation is an analogous ground of discrimination prohibited under s. 15 of the Charter. Gays and lesbians form a historically disadvantaged group, and s. 159 violates s. 15(1) of the Charter because it arbitrarily disadvantages individuals in that historically disadvantaged group -- gay men -- by denying to them until they are 18 a choice available at the age of 14 to those who are not gay, namely, their choice of sexual expression with a consenting partner to whom they are not married. Anal intercourse is a basic form of sexual expression for gay men. The prohibition of this form of sexual conduct in s. 159 accordingly has an adverse impact on them. Section 159 infringes s. 15(1) of the Charter on the grounds of sexual orientation.

The Crown advanced, as a legislative objective sufficiently

pressing and substantial to justify overriding the constitutionally protected right, the objective of protecting young persons from engaging in a specific form of sexual activity, anal intercourse, for which there are increased risks of physical and psychological harm, and, in particular, the increased risk for the transmission of HIV. It is difficult to imagine a more intrusive way to protect an individual from harm than criminal prosecution. Far from minimally impairing the right to equality, the loss of liberty for a consensual form of sexual expression is the most restrictive means possible for achieving the objective. It is inappropriate to deal with minimizing health risks at any age by using the punitive force of the Criminal Code, but especially so for young people.

The measures chosen in s. 159 to protect young people from risk are arbitrary and unfair, compared to the measures used to protect against the health risks for individuals who prefer other forms of sexual conduct. There is no rational connection between protecting someone from the potential harm of exercising sexual preferences and imprisoning that individual for exercising them. There is no proportionality between the articulated health objectives and the draconian criminal means chosen to achieve them. The infringement of s. 15 was not justified under s. 1 of the Charter.

Per Goodman and Catzman JJ.A.: Section 159 of the Criminal Code constitutes an infringement of s. 15 on the ground of age. On the question whether the discriminatory effect of s. 159 can be justified under s. 1 of the Charter, the portion of the reasons of Abella J.A. concluding that s. 159 cannot be so justified are agreed with.

APPEAL by the Crown from a judgment of Corbett J. (1992), 1992 CanLII 12798 (ON SC), 11 C.R.R. (2d) 363,

75 C.C.C. (3d) 556, 15 C.R. (4th) 368 (Gen. Div.),
<u>acquitting the accused on a charge of anal intercourse.</u>

After reading the above court case , do you think
that justice was served for that abuse underage girl?
Was the judge's decision correct or even fair?
Although I am not a lawyer or a judge, I think the
judge ignored the fact that the young girl was
manipulate and sexually abused by an older man
for many years.
I have no idea how the judges make their decision,
but I read in the papers that quite a few judges
made wrong decisions . Like another case
where a woman complaint that she was raped and
reported him to the police. At the time of the trial
the presiding judge let the man free and blamed
the woman why she did not keep her legs closed.
The media and other people were upset by this
particular judge's decision and made a big noise
about that decision. The judge was finally forced
to resign. That proves that judges are human too
and can make mistake with their decisions.
Nobody is infallible no matter what is their
background , education or what position the hold
in society.

Conclusion

In conclusion, anal sex is a highly risky activity which exposes those involved in a huge health risks including sterility. In writing this book I tried to emphasize the fact that ANAL SEX is a sexual abuse of a non sexual organ with potential huge health risks . The use of the anus for sexual activity for a fleetly pleasure and huge health risk makes no sense. But humans are well known for doing things that make no sense and when they suffer the consequences, sometimes they plead ignorance, that they did not know that such an activity would have such a catastrophic effect on their health.

This book is about raising the alarm about the catastrophic effects will have on humanity if everyone starts practicing anal sex for pleasure. Who is going to have babies for the future generations? Anal sex can cause sterility and other diseases to both men and women. The human race might be wiped out of the face of earth. Proponents of the anal sexual abuse, because that's exactly what it is , a sexual abuse of a non sexual organ, emphasize pleasure and more pleasure of such activity, mostly to the perpetrators and ignore the serious health risks to both parties involved. Life is not always about pleasure at any cost, life is about living a healthy life and avoid any potential risks that can put your health and your life in danger. People always have a choice and some people make good choices and some people make bad choices and they pay the price with their health. People are free to make their own choices.

EPILOGUE

Whatever consenting adults are doing in the privacy of their homes is their own business and nobody's else.

In this book I sound the alarm that anal sex is the sexual abuse of a non sexual organ with potential catastrophic consequences on the human health. Whether anal sex is practiced by consenting adults, or non consenting people, the potential health risks are huge and even life threatening. Many people including many youngsters , male and females are sexually abused every year ruining their lives. And that's a big problem for society.

The way things go, anal sexual abuse is spreading like a wild fire and if everyone starts practicing anal sex , the human race might disappear from the face of the earth like SODOM and GOMORRAH. A few thousand years ago, the practice of sodomy put an end to those two sin cities and the wide spread of sodomy in modern times, might put an end to the human race on earth…. That would be the nature's punishment for violating the nature's laws.

References

1)://www.medicalnewstoday.com/articles/156549.php
Anal cancer is a tumor that grows in the anus or **anal** canal. It is a rare form of cancer that tends to be more common in women than men. Risk factors include infection with the human papilloma ...
2)A rare, but serious, complication after anal sex is a hole (perforation) in the colon. This dangerous problem requires hospitalization, surgery to repair the hole, and antibiotics to prevent infection.
3)The research, published in the **medical** journal BMJ Open, attempted to collect information about when **anal sex** occurs and the reasons why men and women engage in it.
Author: Kristen Sollee

*4)https://www.dw.com/en/polands-catholic-**church**-admits-**clergy**...*

News Poland's Catholic **Church** admits **clergy sexually abused** hundreds of **children**. Poland's Catholic **Church** has released a report admitting hundreds of clergymen **abused children** …

*5)https://www.smalljoys.tv/illinois-priests-**abusing-children***

Illinois Attorney General has issued a damning report about **clergy sexual abuse** on Wednesday, saying that the names of more than 500 **clergy** accused of **sexually abusing children** haven't yet released by the state's Catholic dioceses.

Book description:

This book is about the controversial issue of anal sex.

The proponents of this controversial sexual activity , talk about sexual pleasure and more pleasure, but is it worth the potential health risks?

Read this book before you decide if you should

or you should not engage in this controversial sexual activity or any other sexual activity.

 Whatever consenting adults do or do not do in the privacy of their homes, it is their business and nobody's else.

After reading this book,   whatever the readers decide to do or not do , it is their own decision and nobody's else..

 This book is about raising the awareness of the benefits, if any, and mostly the potential   health risks of such a controversial sexual activity.

Any sexual activity is a health issue with many potential health risks.

Anal sex is the abuse of a non sexual organ with potential huge health risks to both parties involved but as long as consenting adults want to take such risks that's their choice and if their health pays the price............well, it is their own choice..

Read the book and make your own decision!

The author.

www.ingramcontent.com/pod-product-compliance
Lightning Source LLC
Chambersburg PA
CBHW031923170526
45157CB00008B/3026